Manageable Fitness
For Women

By Roxanne Eyler

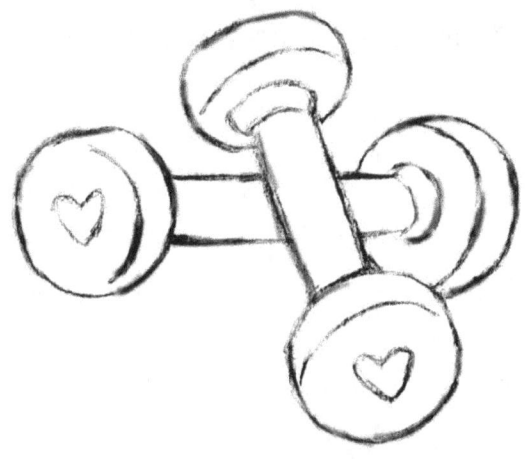

ROXANNE-EYLER.COM

Design by Melissa D. Jones
rouxroamer.com

Illustrations by Melissa Kojima
melissakojima.com

Disclaimer and/or Legal Notices

I am not a doctor and this is not meant to be taken as medical advice.

The information provided in this book is based upon my life experiences along with my interpretations of the available current research.

The advice and tips given in this course are meant for healthy adults, wanting to achieve better fitness. Consult your physician to confirm the tips given in this manual are appropriate for you.

If you have any health issues or pre-existing conditions, please consult with or ask your physician before implementing any of the information provided in this course.

This product is for informational purposes only and the author does not accept any responsibilities for any liabilities or damages, real or perceived, resulting from the use of this information.

Table of Contents

Who Am I?

I am Roxanne Eyler. These are my credentials:
- I have a Bachelor of Science Degree
- C.Ph.T = Certified Pharmacy Technician
- I am a Certified Personal trainer
- I am Certified in FMS The Functional Movement System
- I am AFAA certified in Group Exercise
- I hold a First Degree Black Belt in Mixed Martial Arts

My passion and focus is working with everyday people like myself, and spreading the message and knowledge that balanced fitness can be achieved in a manageable time frame. The one problem I have discovered with most people that are not seeing long-term results, is many people go to the gym and just workout, no program. The answer is you need a program.

Manageable Fitness for Women is one program that will work.

There are one hundred sixty eight hours in the week. Forty of those hours are typically spent working or caring for your family during the day or evening. On average another fifty-six hours are sleeping. Approximately seventy-two hours are left to spend and do whatever you want. Out of those seventy-two hours if you are willing to devote three hours a week you can achieve balanced fitness.

I will show you a program that you can maintain for life. I have created a program that is manageable. This program will not leave you so sore that in two days you're not sure you can do it again. It will leave you feeling like you did something good for yourself, it will leave you feeling accomplished.

I do not believe in diets. Who can maintain a diet for their whole life? If you diet, lose weight and then return to your old eating patterns you will watch the weight creep back on. The combination of using free weights or dumbbells in conjunction with cardiovascular exercise for your workout keeps the program to a manageable time frame of three hours per week. The Manageable Fitness program will help you develop strength and definition to your muscles while also gaining a benefit of increased calorie burn. Proper nutrition will help you to lose weight faster and reshape your body as you move through this fitness program.

Do you want to feel better? Look good in your clothes? Then, keep reading!

If you are looking for 20 percent body fat, six packs abs or some magic formula stop reading now.

This program is structured for average every day people. This is not a program for elite athletes who train six or eight hours a day. I cannot guarantee you will look like a model as the months roll along but you will feel better. To lose weight you will need to make some nutritional changes with the weight and cardio program to further increase your weight loss. Utilizing the program will change the way you look and feel about you, the nutrition changes will increase weight loss.

This program is for average everyday people like me and you, who want to feel good, move better and look good in our clothes and don't have the time to work out endless hours.

Please understand that this program is not a quick, one time fix. You must continue to exercise, do cardio and perform range of motion exercises. The program is like a relationship; something to nurture, to nurture you. You will love the feeling of accomplishment, along with looking and feeling better, and moving better. You can include in your schedule only three hours per week to look and feel great. The other one hundred and sixty five hours are yours to do as you please.

The difference between success and failure is Persistence. When you see someone who looks good, healthy and seems fit, it's not something that happened overnight. They have been persistent in their efforts. As you continue to persist with your workouts, commit to making nutritional changes. Be persistent in your efforts. Nothing happens overnight. One day you may notice that your clothes are feeling bigger or fitting differently. That you are moving better, and that you feel more stable, that your posture has improved. Persistence brings results for your efforts and will further increase your motivation.

Warm up and Resets

The Warm up will mimic the movements we will do and get the muscles ready to do the work. It is not necessary to do a long warm up before you start your work out. For this reason I will have you engage your posterior chain (back side) along with your anterior chain (front side) of your body. All muscles and ligaments in our body are connected and need to work together; we are a giant X. When we connect all parts of the body it helps us to prevent injury. It also strengthens the entire body allowing it to work together and helps the other muscles that are doing the direct work. One example of how this works: If we are performing an overhead shoulder press. Give this a try.

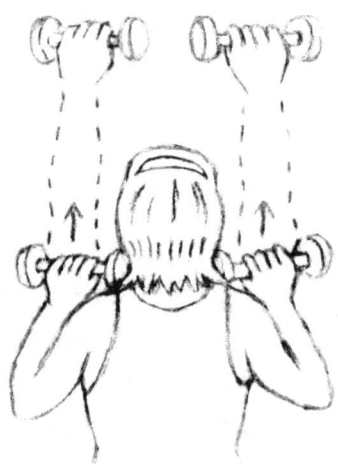

We want to roll our shoulders back and down so that our shoulders are connected to (shoulder and side muscles) our lats or latissimus dorsi along with the rhomboids and scapula. These muscles will all work together to provide more strength and will help other muscles when performing the exercises. Use the illustration above and when you perform the movement you can feel how all of these muscles are working together. Knowing how to properly align your body and linking (connecting) everything together allows all of the muscles and ligaments to work together helping to prevent injury and allowing for greater strength in the movement. Performing the exercises without linking and connecting your muscles for the movement increases your chance of injury over time.

Getting Started

Range of motion exercises will improve mobility and help with some of the simple movements we do in everyday life. For example if you drive a car you need to be able to look over your shoulder to change lanes, or maybe at home you need to squat down to pick up an item. We need to be able to perform movement in life without injury. The range of motion exercises I will give you can simply be done in the shower if you want that's where I do them, or any other time or place that is convenient. I will list a few range of motion exercises with the warm ups and resets in the next chapter. Foam rolling can also be part of a warm up to release tension, get some blood flow in the muscle and loosen the fascia around your muscles.

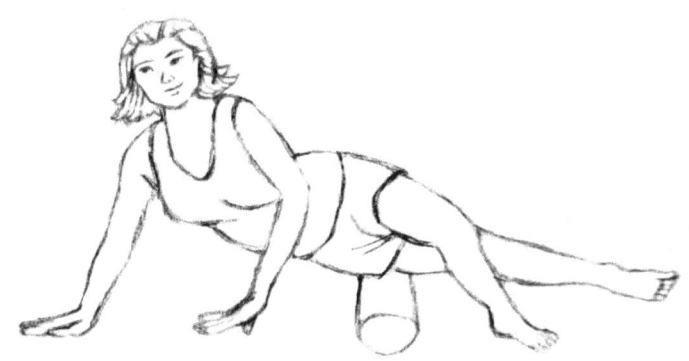

Exercises for Range of Motion

You can perform the range of motion exercises in any order you like. Perform at least five repetitions of the following five movements.

1. Neck Nods

The basic neck nod can be done on all fours or you may do this standing if you prefer.

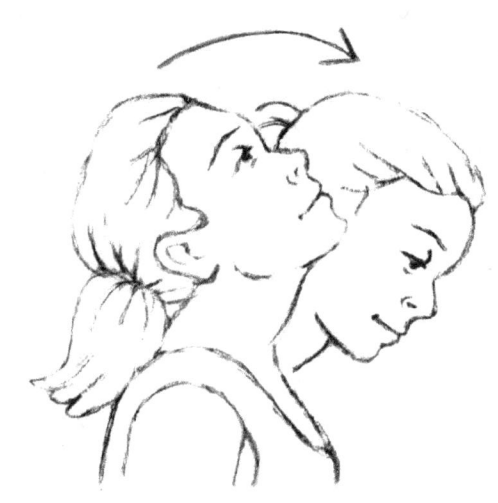

Simply look down slowly and tuck your chin to your chest then look up slowly with your eyes and lift your head. Repeat several times. At first you may find that your neck seems tight don't worry it will loosen up as you perform the exercise.

2. Looking Side to Side

Standing with your hands down by your sides roll shoulders back and look to your left and try to get your chin in line up with your shoulder then back to center and now go to your right.

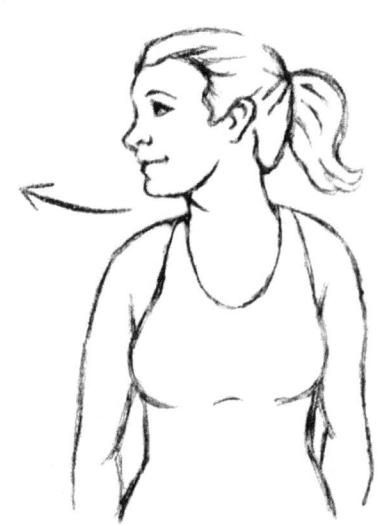

Remember to complete at least five reps. (Center-right-center-left = one rep)

3. Ear to Shoulder Tilt

Stand straight with your shoulders rolled back and down. Gently tilt your head to the side and let your ear drop toward your

Shoulder, hold for a few seconds then back to center. Do this stretch on both sides.

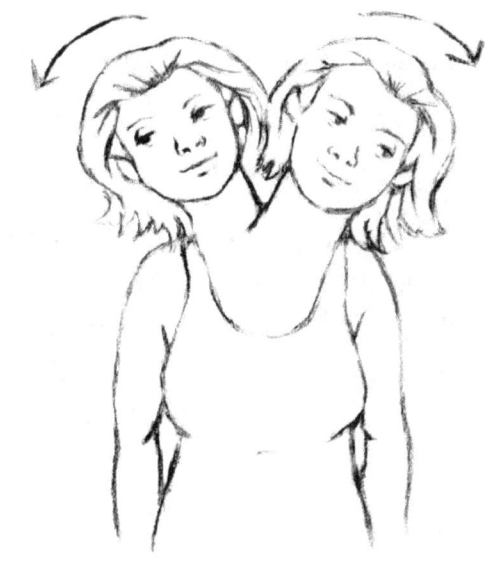

4. Reach Behind/Side Reach

Standing with feet shoulder width apart or sitting, roll shoulders back and down. Take your right hand and reach to your left, let your left hand start to rotate behind you. While looking at your right hand, let your eyes look farther behind and try to reach farther than where you are currently looking. Where the head and eyes go, the body follows. Look beyond where you are reaching. Do this on both sides of your body.

You can get more mobility or more movement in your thoracic spine also known as the upper part of your back doing this exercise. Sitting upright fold arms over Indian style, now turn to one side as far as you can, now tip arms down, you should feel that stretch. Do this on both sides five times.

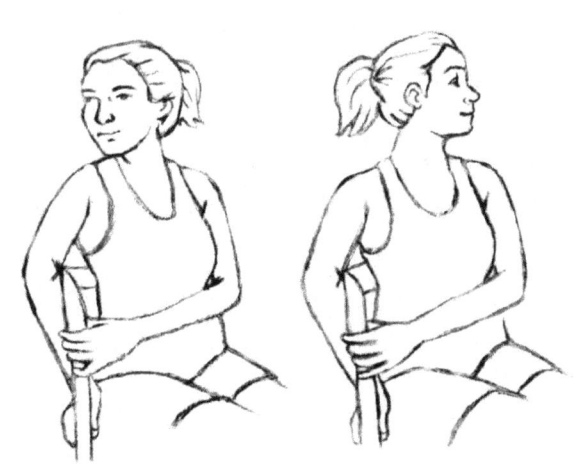

5. Circles, Arms, Hands, Knees, Feet, Hips

There is no set number have fun with this. The movements help to get synovial fluid in your joints.

This movement is done standing. Make big circles with your arms, then your hands, put your knees together and make circles with them. While standing lift a foot off the floor and make circles. This foot circle exercise can even be done lying in bed. I do foot circles in bed before I get up. Then make some circles with your hips.

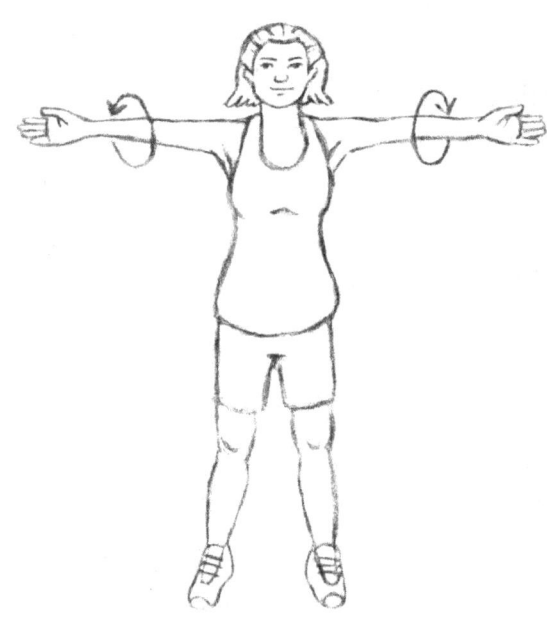

Movement Resets

Movement resets help you to regain your normal movement patterns. Normal movement patterns connect both sides of our body communicating with each other to help with our balance and normal walking gait.

As we go through life the turned ankles, falls or daily activities affect our bodies. We may not realize it but our bodies automatically compensate for these happenings and may change our movement pattern. Compensations by our body is done to protect the injured area and help out the knee, or ankle that might have been hurt. We may slip, fall, lift something too heavy, and sit for long periods of time, garden or simply lack movement in our life. All of the above affects our posture possibly creating a forward shoulder roll (getting that hump in your back) lower back stiffness, or inability to look over our shoulder when we drive.

The following small movements or "resets" will help you to regain what you may not know you lost. I recommend doing them as frequently as possible.

Movement resets can be done before working out, after or any other time. Making sure you do them is what is important. Resets can also be done and will help on days you are not working out. The small time investment of five to ten minutes will be well worth it.

Rocking

Babies know what they are doing.

Rocking is how babies gain their core strength and teach both sides of the brain to communicate with one another, by rocking. If you can get on all fours, look forward and try to have the crown (top) of your head pointing up towards the ceiling. Now push yourself back towards your feet (keep looking forward) then rock forward all while trying to keep the crown (top) of your head up toward the ceiling.

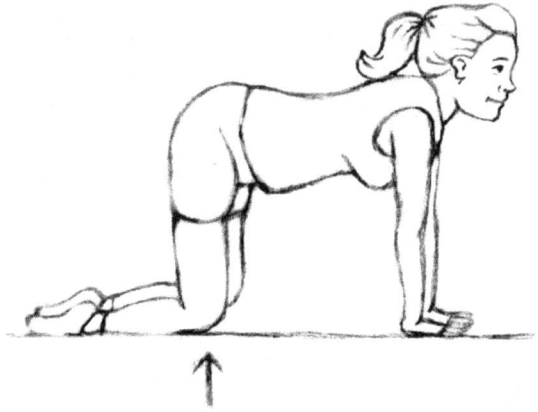

Rolling

You may start on your stomach or back. Rolling can be done on the floor or if you cannot get down on the floor your bed can suffice. Starting from your back, reach up overhead with your arms. Now take both arms and bring it up overhead as in the picture below. To begin to roll, reach across your body without using your leg for momentum and continue to roll until you run out of space. Look ahead of your hand with your eyes.

Do this on both sides. Then try it using your legs now. It may be difficult at first, but make sure your eyes follow or look ahead of where you want to go. Where your eyes look, your body will follow. We know what we are doing from the moment we are born to gain strength and movement we just lose it over time due to lifestyle or life incidents we encounter.

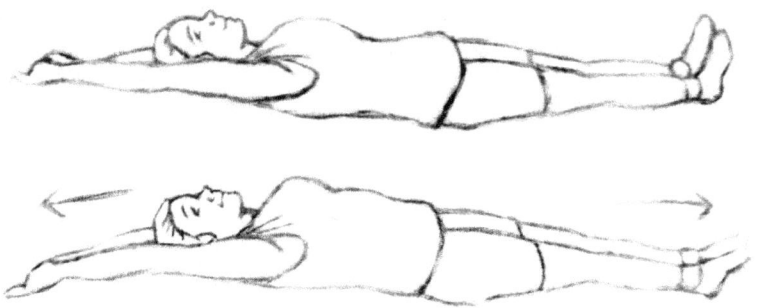

Original Strength is a book written by Geoff Neupert and Tim Anderson. The book has been an exceptional resource for my clients and me. These exercises are from that book and I use these myself. I have had clients with very tight hip flexors gain more mobility using these exercises. One client in his 50's was so pulled forward from tight hip flexors he was having back issues and gaining a forward shoulder roll. Implementing these movements and cross patterns as well as the posterior and anterior chain movements helped to free and loosen up his hip flexors bringing him more upright and moving better.

The book utilizes marching or cross patterns as well as rocking to reset the vestibular system, which is the mind body connection, and to reset movement and posture. These movements will help you gain strength. The basis of the book in a short snippet, is that babies know exactly how to build strength and movement so we emulate these movements to get our movement patterns and strength back. This is where we started and this is where we start. Getting on all fours (if possible) on the ground looking forward, chest open and rocking like a small child does before they walk. Now, we can move on to the exercises. Before we do, there are a few rules. For moving and lifting the weights.

Rule 1

I will explain to you how to keep your posterior chain and anterior chain linked. This must be practiced and utilized for each and every exercise. The weights we move from rows to presses and lateral raises, everything must be linked this is the most important rule.

Rule 2

We are not going to tear that muscle to gain strength and size. We want strength and definition. As you go through the five sets of five reps if at any point, possibly in the third or fourth rep of the fifth set, you struggle to move that weight. Don't do that rep.

When you build muscle it is called hypertrophy. There are different types of hypertrophy and we want to practice the kind that develops strength and definition, not size. My opinion is that most women would like to look toned and defined so this is how we will proceed, 5 x 5 without tearing the muscle and lifting heavy.

Posterior and Anterior Chain Linking

Sean Schniederjan has books out that I use in my practice on how to keep the body connected by linking your posterior and anterior chain. First to link the posterior chain, stand straight with your hands by your sides. Roll your shoulders back and down. Now, drive your heels into the floor. As you drive your heels into the floor it's ok if your toes come up off the floor a little. You should feel your hamstrings (back of your legs) start to engage; your glutes (butt) engaged and feel the tension moving up your back. Keep pressing those heels into the floor now for the anterior; squeeze your abs like someone is going to hit you in the stomach with a board or fat uncle is going to come and sit on you.

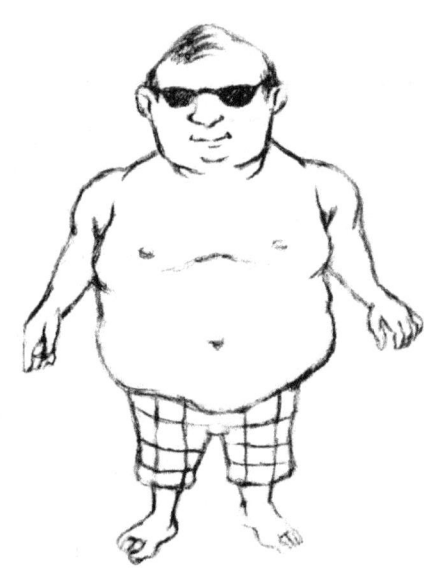

Now, make believe you are pulling a weight into your chest. You now have everything linked. That is how it should feel when you're doing the exercises. If you link your posterior and anterior chain, then even without a weight in hand you can create demand on the muscle and it will feel like you are moving a weight.

Heels driven into the floor, shoulders down and back, abs really pulled in and tight.

Now, as your arms are down by your side, palms facing in, squeeze the sides of your chest with your arm and make believe you are curling a dumbbell up. You start with palms facing in by your side, but as you raise your arms turn palms up toward the sky when you reach waist height, then continue to raise the weight to chest level. Without any weight in your hand because your have done this linked, under tension you should feel this in your biceps. The process of linking, connecting and keeping tension while performing the exercise movement with the weight is similar to how an isometric movement is done.

Now that you have been introduced to how to best do the exercises, we can start the workouts. The exercises and sheets describing them have been set up so that they can be printed out and taken to the gym or wherever you workout.

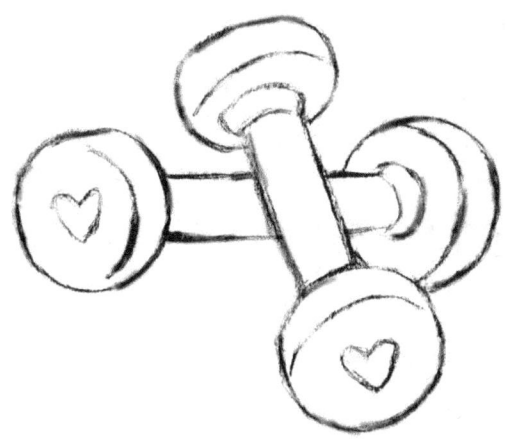

Day 1 — 5 sets of 5

ONE ARM DUMBBELL (DB) ROW
Knee on bench one foot on floor. Get linked. Extend one arm out all the way then pull or row with arm by side up with elbow toward sky.

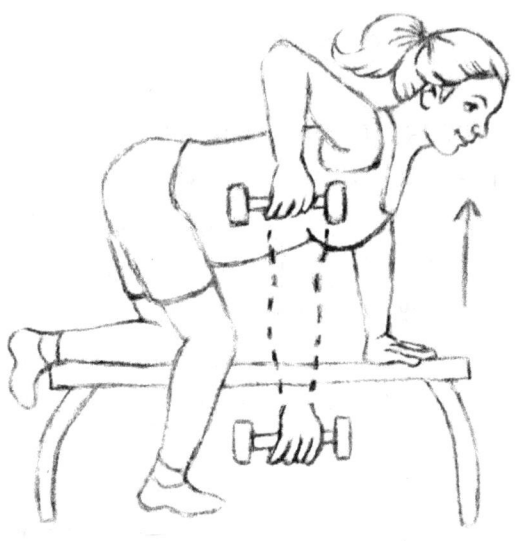

DUMBBELL PULLOVER
Lying on a flat bench with feet on floor or bench, head at end with DB. Extend dumbbell above chest return to start.

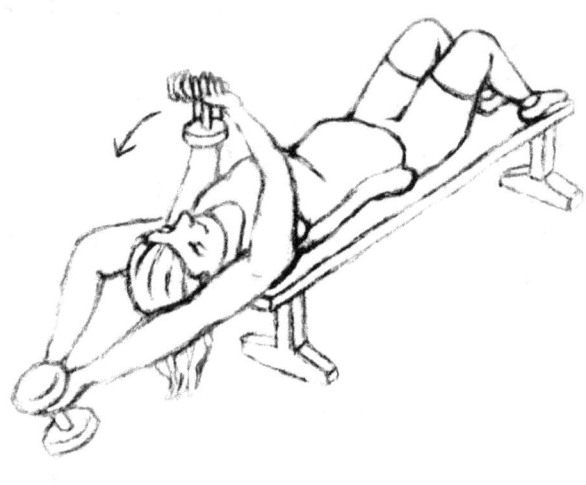

DUMBBELL FLY
Arms outstretched to side, palms facing in, slight bend in elbows. Bring DB together like your hugging a barrel. On bench or floor change up on day 1 & 3.

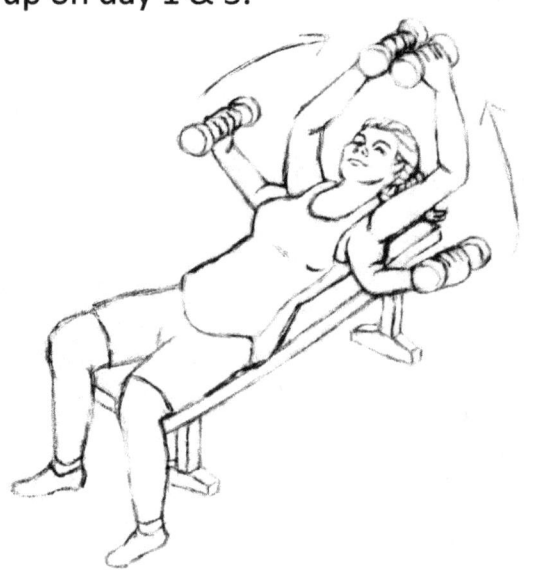

DB PRESS-STANDING
Start DB palms out, shoulder height. GET Linked. Drive weights straight overhead, do not lock out elbows, bring back down to shoulder height.

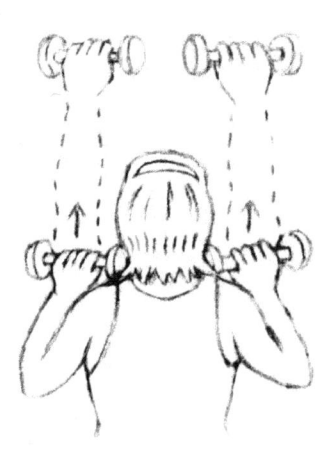

PLANK–FOREARMS OR HANDS

Begin lying on floor, face down elbows underneath your shoulders, come up on your toes and elbows push yourself up into plank and hold as long as you can. Can be done on knees.

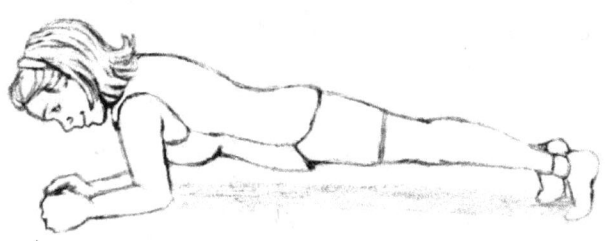

DEAD BUGS

Back on floor, bring arms and legs up together, alternate opposite arm and leg together lowering to the ground and back to start.

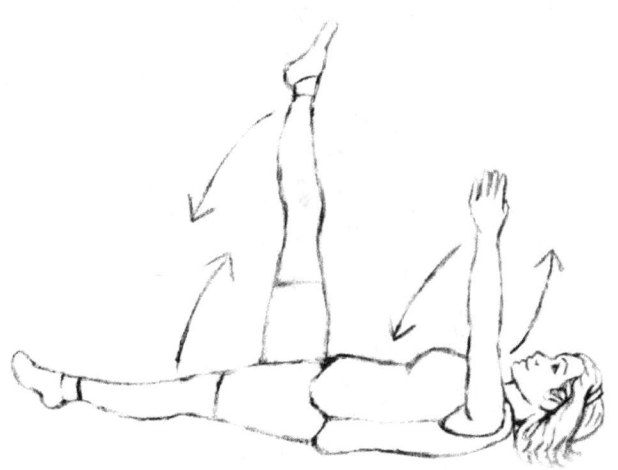

Day 2 — 5 sets of 5

SEATED DUMBBELL PRESS

Start DB palms out shoulder height. Push feet into the floor. Get linked. Drive weights straight overhead, do not lock out elbows, bring back down to shoulder height.

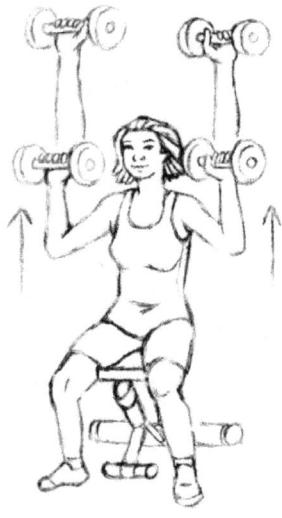

DB LATERAL RAISE

Stand palms facing in with DB's in hands. Push feet into ground (getting linked) roll shoulders down and back raise arms to shoulder height and return to start position.

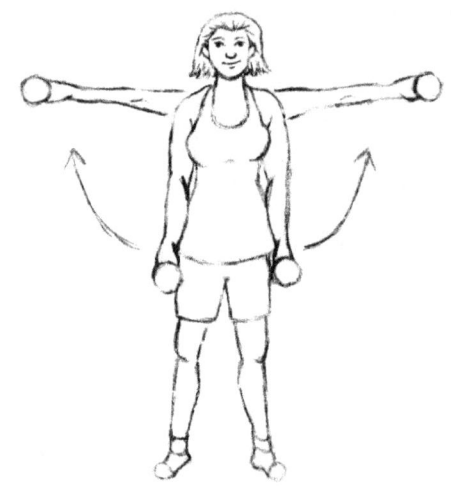

SEATED DB CURLS

Sit on bench. DB in each hand, palms facing in. Curl one arm at a time rotate wrist hip high so palms face up, return to start, fully extend arms out.

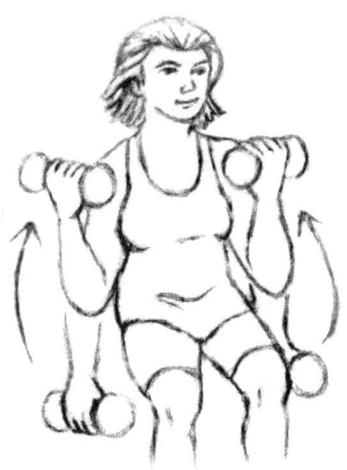

CONCENTRATION CURL

Sit on bench, feet on ground, bend over with DB in one hand, palm facing up, elbow touching inside of thigh. Slowly raise hand up toward other arm and back down. Alternate arms.

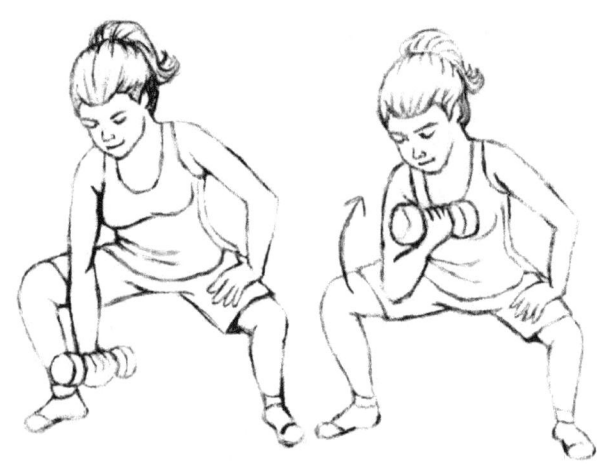

SEATED DB TRICEP EXT.

On bench lower DB behind head with both hands, drive DB up overhead, pause, return to start. Get linked, pushing feet into the floor.

TRICEP DB KICKBACKS

Lean forward, place one arm on bench or knee for support. Arm should be in "L" position. Extend elbow and push DB behind you, return to start.

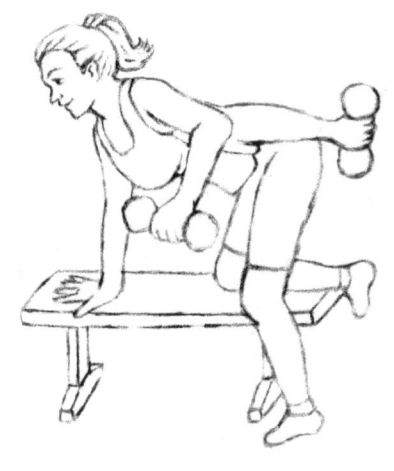

Day 3 — 5 sets of 5

LYING LEG RAISES 20X3

Back on bench or floor turn palms toward ceiling. Push your back into the bench or ground and raise legs, pause at top, lower legs. Can be done bent leg, it's easier.

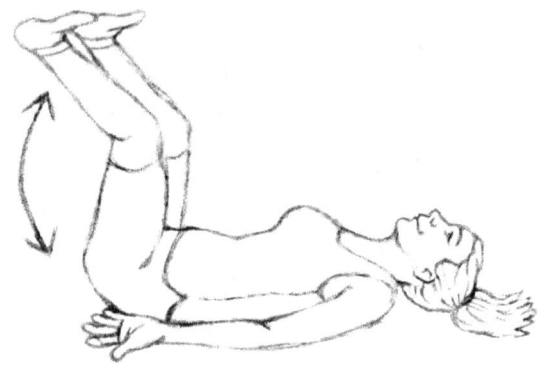

PLANK UP TO 3 MIN

Start by holding for 30 seconds or as long as possible. Keep trying until you can get to holding a 3 minute plank. Forearms or hands, squeeze glutes & stomach.

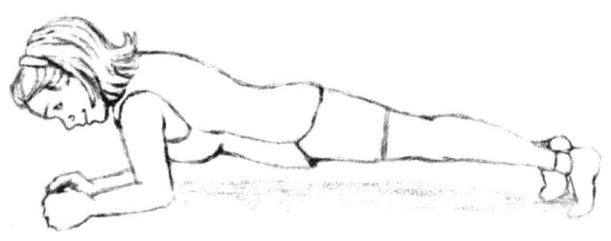

CHOP & LIFT BANDS

From a kneeling, upright position. Band position is above shoulder, overhand. Start a chopping action by pulling in to chest and down across body. Lift band position is low. Start overhand position pull into chest and lower hand up across body to toward shoulder.

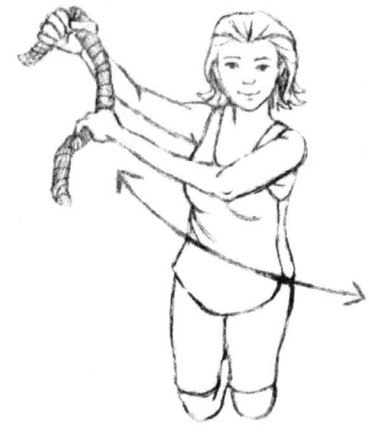

DB FLY INCLINED

Arms outstretched to sides, palms facing in, slight bend in elbows. Bring arms together like you're hugging a barrel. Position is opposite of day one. Get linked.

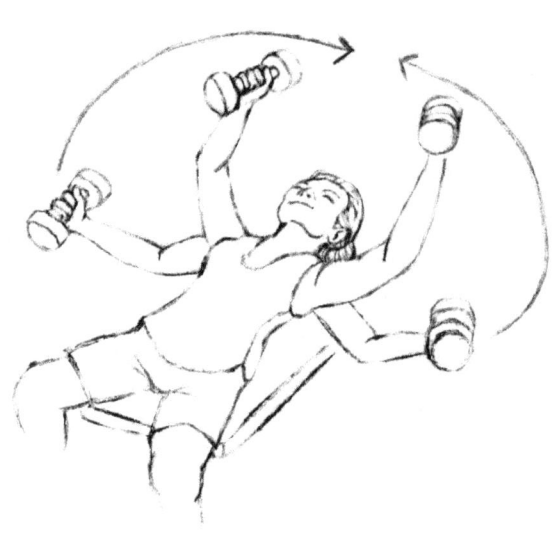

SEATED DB PRESS

Start DB palms out, shoulder height. Get linked. Drive weights straight overhead do not lock out elbows, bring back down to start.

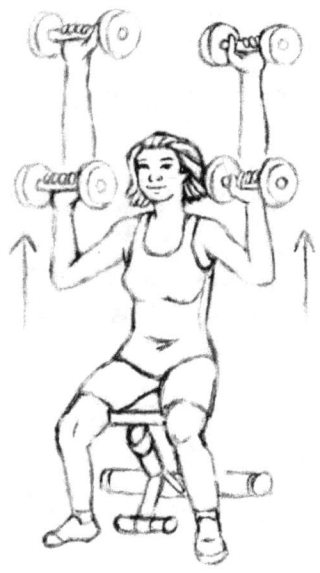

OVERHEAD DB EXT

Sitting or standing, place hands on DB one over the top of other. Extend DB over head. Start behind head and extend up, elbows close. Get Linked.

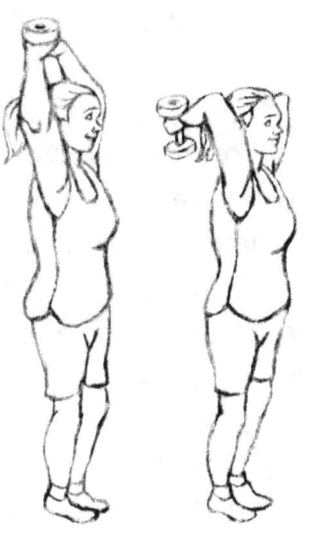

I chose Dumbbells (DB) because they are readily available. These exercises can be done with a variety of pieces of equipment: bands, kettle bells, and sandbags. Use a machine at the gym or a different piece of equipment doing the same exercises once a month to give your body a change and keep some muscle confusion involved in the process.

Here are the rules:

1. Remember all exercises are done LINKED and under TENSION.
2. Do not try to be a hero and kill yourself lifting as much as possible or cheat yourself by not using enough weight or tension.
3. Find the correct weight that you can use and move through each exercise without failure (maybe a little struggle when you get to that last set). You should feel tired and it should feel hard but do not break down and tear the muscle to failure. Write down your weight, 10lb or whichever you use, for each exercise. Then you don't have to remember.
4. Do not perform the rep if you have reached failure in that set. Here's an example: if you are struggling during your fourth set when you get to the third, fourth or fifth repetition do only three reps, or four, whatever you can get out. Take a break and move on to the last set doing as many as you can.
5. You will not change the size of your weight until after completing five reps of five sets seems easy. Only then you should increase or move up the size of the weight.
6. You should not feel that two day on set soreness. You should feel as though you worked out but not so sore you don't want to workout again.
7. Find a friend to workout with. This can keep you both going, motivated and supported. It's good to have a support network.

The sets above are the lifting program. This should take about 25 minutes.

You must also do 30 minutes of cardio, following your weights, never before you do weights. You will do interval cardio. Examples would be running: 30 seconds running (work hard) then 30 seconds walking. Do those for 15 minutes then walk at a steady state for 15 minutes following your interval. You can do this on a treadmill, fast and slow walking, elliptical at the gym or a bike. For the first 15 minutes you want to elevate your heart rate up and down, then do a steady pace for the balance of time. You can lengthen and shorten your interval time. Minute on minute slow as your endurance becomes better. Now you have the basic program.

Every three months it would be good to change your routine. This will add variety along with improving your workout. You can change this by using cabled machines at the gym, changing the speed you move the weights, using machines for a month. Your workout can be changed weekly by also changing the speed that you move the weights: using a lighter one than your regular routine and moving it faster or you can use the same weight or a little heavier weight and slow down the movement. Variety truly is the spice of life and keeps you progressing and interested with some variety in your workout.

Foam Rolling

Foam rolling is a great way to give yourself a massage to get some blood flow back in the muscle. Foam rolling can be a great asset before and after workouts. The Internet has various resources and videos on foam rolling it's very simple, although it may seem awkward at first. Give it a try.

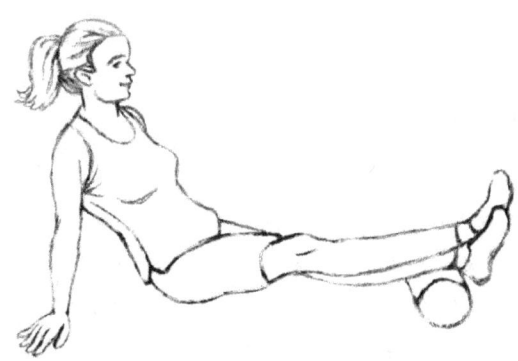

Nutrition

Nutrition is one of the key factors in weight loss. If you would like to lose weight, you must adhere to the nutritional aspect of the program. Success is 60-80 percent dependent on your nutrition. Exercise cannot make up for poor nutrition. Let me emphasize, this is not a diet but I would like you to start looking at the foods you eat and pay attention to the additives in the food you are eating. Begin to explore the idea of more whole foods. If it's on the label and you cannot pronounce it or have no idea what it is, you might want to make a different food choice. Considering the decisions on your food choices works better than drastic calorie cutting. Grass fed beef; chicken, organic vegetables and fruits should be the basis of your diet. If you do not feel ready to start buying organic at least try to incorporate more whole foods into your life. Then do the research so you know why grass fed and organic is better.

An excellent place to start is Foodbabe.com. This website has a wealth of excellent information and recipes. The food babe reveals additives such as the petroleum (yep, same stuff that's in your car) in food and, beaver butt (yes beaver butt) that is used as a natural flavor instead of the actual flavors. Is this good or bad? Natural sounds good but is it?

Got your attention? Right! No one probably chooses to eat beaver butt, so why does the FDA allow that in our food? It is not necessary to run out and go all organic or vegan but it is important to be informed about the additives and other suspect substances that makes it's way into the food we eat. The problem is these additives effect how our bodies' respond or the hormonal response by our body when ingested many times preventing us from losing weight. Our brain may not be getting the satiety or fullness signal; maybe glucose in our body is affected. Food additives, or the products manufacturers add to packaged food can cause ADHD, allergies, migraines as well as many other problems or complications. Be informed about your food choices, so you know what you want to choose.

Ezekiel bread is a regular staple in my personal diet. Ezekiel bread can, in some instances, be eaten by gluten-intolerant people. Ezekiel bread can be very filling and also contains protein and protein helps to create a feeling of fullness so you may find you eat less. I happen to like free-range eggs. Eggs are an excellent source of protein along with being the only complete food; a complete food is one that has all of your basic nutritional needs. The cholesterol in eggs is the kind of cholesterol our body needs. We will focus more on the nutrition portion as we move along through the book. Most importantly begin to consider what your nutrition looks like.

To lose weight, you may want to create a calorie deficit; one way to do this is fasting. I know fasting may sound scary, stay with me, research shows one good way to create a calorie deficit is to skip breakfast one or two days a week and hold out until lunch or after if you can. Nothing to eat after dinner and then going until lunch time twice per week can easily create a eight or nine hundred calorie deficit. Some people may feel that breakfast is the most important meal of the day, if so try this by eliminating dinner if you are looking to create a fast. That time period of approximately eighteen hours is considered fasting giving your GI tract a break. The fast period creates a calorie deficit by missing breakfast towards the 3500 calories needed to lose a pound of weight. Give it a try if it doesn't interfere with any health concerns you have, which would interfere with missing a meal. Create a routine of small changes only changing one thing at a time. Instead of getting up getting some coffee, tea or soda down right away, whichever your morning beverage might be. Start by hydrating and alkalizing your body. One change that has worked well for me: First thing in the morning before my coffee I drink 8 ounces of lemon water. I squeeze a fresh lemon into a little cold water in a glass then fill the rest with the warmest water I can drink. This is a great way to help alkalize your body, and it is good for your liver and GI system. It helps to keep your GI system clean and functioning properly. Try to make just one small change at a time... nothing dramatic. Each small change adds up to bigger lifestyle changes over time.

Small Changes

I briefly discussed nutrition earlier and the need to not diet but find a way to make small changes for nutritional success. Everyone has different physiological and dietary needs. If you were diabetic you would have a problem incorporating intermittent fasting into your program. If you're diabetic, your weight loss may be a little slower but your numbers after working out for two weeks and forward will start to drop and sometimes dramatically, so always consult with your doctor.

You can keep track of calories and the ratio of protein, fats and carbs with a number of apps such as *Lose It*, *My Fitness Pal* and many others. Look online or through the app source on your phone. There are a number of free resources if you are interested in tracking your calories. These applications will also give you a better understanding, visually, of your nutrition and if you have too many carbs or too many fats in your nutrition plan.

First, starting with basic nutrition please consider giving up all the processed foods that have hidden sugars. There are numerous articles on the Internet citing how addicting high fructose corn syrup is. More addicting than cocaine, HFC is hidden is many processed foods. The hormonal response our bodies have on the additives in food many times prevents us from the success we can achieve by trying to eat cleaner. That doesn't mean you have to give up that dessert or sweet treat forever but consider how much hidden sugar you're actually ingesting.

Calculating the number of calories you should ingest per day can be tiresome. If you are interested in tracking, use one of the online tools available for your phone or computer. As a rule, women should never consume less than 1200 calories per day. If you're not interested in tracking calories you do not have to. Start doing some research on whole foods; grass fed chicken, beef, seafood, organic grains and vegetables. Many recipes are available if you're interested in incorporating a more holistic or organic lifestyle into your fitness regimen. Just remember if you're looking for weight loss it boils down to calories in and calories out no matter what your food selection is. You cannot "out exercise" a bad diet, period. If you are interested in creating a calorie deficit I have outlined below an intermittent fasting routine that you can do once, no more than twice, per week to create a calorie deficit.

To try the 24-hour fast, pick one day this week where you will be free to go 24 hours without food. One option would be to eat dinner the night before, fast throughout the day and have a normal size dinner that night. You may prefer to eat breakfast and then go without food until the next day's breakfast. Ultimately the timing doesn't matter, just go 24 hours without calories.

During the fast it is important to stay hydrated. Try to drink at least 80-102 ounces of water during the day. Black coffee and green tea (another anti inflammatory) is also permitted. Just make sure you're not getting too many calories in your beverages.

Drinking plenty of fluids will also help you curb waves of hunger that will surface and then go away throughout the day. Respond to hunger by taking in more fluids and it will soon pass.

The 24-hour fast is much easier then it sounds and gets even easier the second time around, when you know what to expect. You can partake in one or two 24-hour fasts each week. Don't do any more than two per week.

If you're pregnant or diabetic, fasting in most instances is not right for you. Consult with your doctor before fasting.

If you're ready to burn more fat while drastically improving your health, give fasting a try. Start with the 24-hour fast and see for yourself how relatively painless it can be to do less. (Every subsequent fast gets a little bit easier.)

Persistence = Success

I wanted to close the book by confirming the success that I have had with clients. Many of my clients have successfully increased their mobility, strength and definition along with weight loss. I can show you how to do the exercises, the necessary steps to gain a healthier eating lifestyle, but only you can make these changes.

Visit my blog at Roxanne-eyler.com for testimonials, nutrition tips, recipes and various workouts.

I have struggled with weight due to hormonal issues, and on occasion, too many get-togethers with my friends or not making the better food choices. We all have our ups and downs. I understand the struggle and want to reach as many people as possible to let them know exercise can and does lift your spirits, increase your mobility, strength and health.

This program offers us the opportunity to do the things we want to do, look and feel good along the way in a manageable time frame. This program can be continued forever with small changes or you may want to move on to more complex or difficult programs. This is your life and you get to choose. We are meant to move, hopefully this will keep you moving and progressing.

To your persistence and success in what can easily be incorporated into everyone's life, I wrote this book as a start towards your health and fitness.

Have fun.

CONVENIENT LAMINATED WORK-OUT RINGS

TAKE A DAY WITH YOU FOR YOUR WORKOUT

ORDER ON LINE AT:
ROXANNE-EYLER.COM

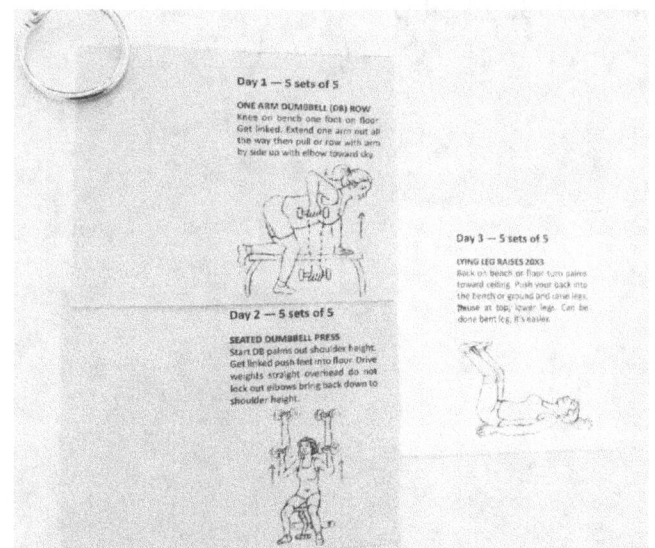

Sources

1. Aksungar F.B. et al. (2007), Interleukin-6, C-Reactive Protein and Biochemical Parameters during Prolonged Intermittent Fasting, Annals of Nutrition and Metabolism,

April 2007, 51:88-95

2. Intermountain Medical Center, http://www.eurekalert.org/pub_releases/2011-04/imc-sfr033111.php